Epilepsy Guide

A family and patient guide on seizures , diagnosis , treatment and more .

CONTENTS

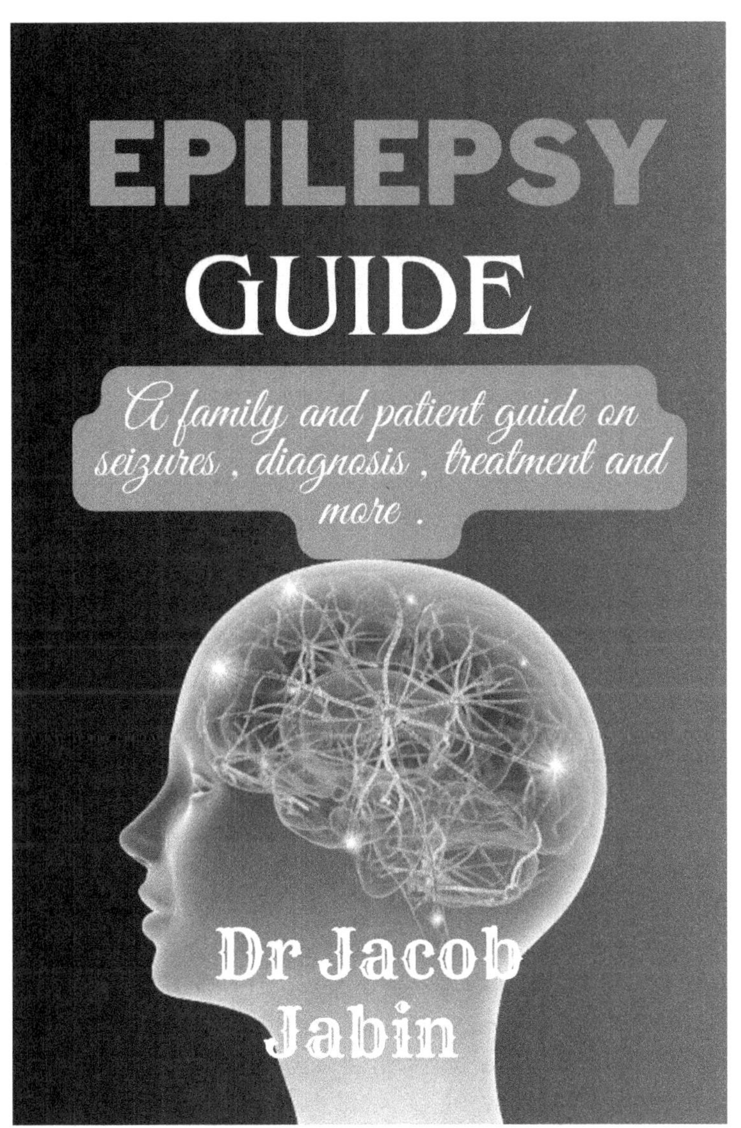

EPILEPSY
GUIDE
A family and patient guide on seizures , diagnosis , treatment and more .
Dr Jacob Jabin

INTRODUCTION

Epilepsy is a neurological illness that affects millions of people throughout the world. It is characterized by repeated and unexpected seizures, which are abrupt bursts of aberrant electrical activity in the brain. Epilepsy may have a substantial influence on the quality of life of patients and their families, since it can create physical, mental, emotional, and social issues. Epilepsy may also be a cause of anxiety, misunderstanding, and stigma, as many people do not understand what it is and how to cope with it.

That is why I developed this book, to present you with accurate, reliable, and up-to-date information about epilepsy, and to help you through the path of living with and managing this illness. I am a neurologist and an epileptologist, which means that I specialize in the diagnosis and treatment of epilepsy. I have more than 20 years of expertise in working with patients and families impacted by epilepsy, and I have watched their challenges and accomplishments. I have also undertaken substantial research and published numerous articles and books on epilepsy, and I have participated in several national and international conferences and seminars on this issue.

In this book, I will share with you my expertise, thoughts, and suggestions on epilepsy, based on the latest scientific facts and best practices. I will also cover some of the frequent issues and worries that you may have, and provide you with practical and realistic solutions and recommendations. I will also offer you emotional and moral support, and urge you to have a positive and proactive approach towards epilepsy.

My major purpose and intention in producing this book is to help you understand and manage epilepsy, and to enable you to live a happy and meaningful life. I hope that this book will give you vital knowledge, practical guidance, and emotional support, and that it will motivate you to embrace and overcome epilepsy.

CHAPTER 1

What is Epilepsy?

Epilepsy is a neurological disorder that affects the brain and causes seizures. A seizure is a rapid and abnormal alteration in the brain's electrical activity, which can impact how a person feels, thinks, behaves, or moves. Seizures can vary in frequency, length, strength, and kind, depending on the source and location of the aberrant brain activity. Some seizures may be minor and scarcely visible, while others may be severe and life-threatening. Some seizures may affect only a region of the brain, while others may impact the complete brain. Some seizures may have a known trigger, such as stress, lack of sleep, or flashing lights, while others may occur without any obvious explanation.

The brain is made of billions of nerve cells, or neurons, that interact with each other through electrical and chemical messages. These signals are responsible for managing all the activities of the body and mind, such as respiration, heartbeat, movement, sensation, memory, emotion, and cognition. Normally, these signals are well-coordinated and balanced, allowing the brain to work smoothly and effectively. However, sometimes, these impulses might become aberrant and disorganized, resulting in a seizure. A seizure can disrupt the normal functioning of the brain and cause various symptoms, such as loss of consciousness, confusion, memory loss, muscle spasms, twitching, jerking, stiffening, shaking, tingling, numbness, vision changes, hearing changes, smell changes, taste changes, mood changes, or hallucinations.

The Causes Of Epilepsy

Epilepsy is diagnosed when a person experiences two or more unprovoked seizures, meaning that they are not triggered by a reversible disease, such as low blood sugar, alcohol withdrawal, or fever. Epilepsy may afflict everyone, regardless of age, gender, color, ethnicity, or origin. According to the World Health Organization (WHO), around 50 million individuals worldwide have epilepsy, making it one of the most common neurological illnesses. Epilepsy may have a substantial influence on the quality of life of patients and their families, since it can create physical, mental, emotional, and social issues. Epilepsy may also be a cause of anxiety, misunderstanding, and stigma, as many people do not understand what it is and how to cope with it.

The specific etiology of epilepsy is not understood in most cases, although it is considered to be a result of a complex combination of genetic, environmental, and biological factors. Some of the probable causes or risk factors of epilepsy include:

- **Genetic factors:** Some kinds of epilepsy are hereditary, meaning that they are handed down from parents to children through genes. Genes are the basic components of heredity that define the qualities and attributes of a person. Some genes can impact the development and function of the brain, and some can make a person more prone to seizures. About 30% to 40% of epilepsy cases are considered to have a hereditary component.

- **Environmental influences:** Some kinds of epilepsy are acquired, meaning that they are produced by external causes that impact the brain. Some of the frequent environmental causes that might induce epilepsy are head trauma, brain infection, brain tumor, stroke, brain malformation, brain inflammation, brain surgery, or exposure to chemicals. These causes can harm or change the structure or function of the brain, and trigger or raise the risk of seizures. About 60% to 70% of epilepsy cases are thought to have an environmental component.

- **Biological considerations:** Some kinds of epilepsy are regulated by internal factors that impact the brain. Some of the typical biological variables that might cause epilepsy are hormone changes, metabolic changes, immune system changes, or neurotransmitter abnormalities. These variables can influence or disturb the balance or control of the brain's electrical and chemical activity, and affect the seizure threshold or frequency. These variables can also interact with genetic or environmental factors, and enhance or reduce the susceptibility or severity of epilepsy.

Types Of Epilepsy Seizures

Epilepsy is not a single disease, but a spectrum of disorders that have varied causes, forms, and presentations. There are various methods to define epilepsy, but one of the most generally used classifications is based on the International League Against Epilepsy (ILAE) classification, which divides epilepsy into three primary categories: focal epilepsy, generalized epilepsy, and unknown epilepsy.

- **Focal epilepsy:** Focal epilepsy, also known as partial epilepsy, is the most prevalent kind of epilepsy, accounting for around 60% of all cases. Focal epilepsy occurs when the seizures originate from a single location or region of the brain, termed the focus. The focus can be positioned in any section of the brain, such as the temporal lobe, the frontal lobe, the parietal lobe, or the occipital lobe. The symptoms and effects of focal epilepsy depend on the function and location of the focus, and might vary from person to person. Focal epilepsy can be further classified into two subtypes:

focal aware seizures and focal impaired awareness seizures.

- Focal aware seizures: Focal aware seizures, also known as simple partial seizures, are seizures that do not impact the knowledge or consciousness of the person. The individual stays conscious and aware of what is occurring throughout the seizure, and can remember it afterwards. Focal aware seizures can elicit numerous sensory, motor, or psychological symptoms, such as tingling, numbness, twitching, jerking, stiffening, shaking, visual changes, hearing changes, smell changes, taste changes, mood changes, or hallucinations. Focal conscious seizures normally last for a few seconds to a few minutes, and do not require any medical intervention.

- Focal impaired awareness seizures: Focal impaired awareness seizures, also known as complex partial seizures, are seizures that influence the awareness or consciousness of the person. The person becomes confused, bewildered, or ignorant of what is occurring during the seizure, and may not recall it afterwards. Focal impaired awareness seizures can elicit numerous behavioral, cognitive, or emotional symptoms, such as gazing, blinking, lip smacking, chewing, swallowing, fidgeting, roaming, muttering, laughing, sobbing, or terror. Focal impaired awareness seizures normally persist for a few minutes, and may require medical intervention.

- Generalized epilepsy: Generalized epilepsy, also known as primary epilepsy, is a kind of epilepsy that develops when the seizures encompass the full brain, rather than a specific location or region. Generalized epilepsy is less prevalent than focal epilepsy, accounting for roughly 40% of all occurrences. Generalized epilepsy is typically caused by hereditary reasons, and often begins in infancy or adolescence. The signs and consequences of generalized epilepsy are largely identical for most people, and can affect both sides of the body and mind. Generalized epilepsy can be further split into six subtypes: absence seizures, tonic seizures, clonic seizures, tonic-clonic seizures, atonic seizures, and myoclonic seizures.

- Absence seizures: Absence seizures, also known as petit mal seizures, are seizures that induce a transient and rapid loss of awareness or consciousness. The person looks to be looking blankly into space, and may not respond to any stimulation. Absence seizures normally last for a few seconds, and might occur multiple times a day. Absence seizures are more prevalent in children than in adults, and can interfere with learning and concentration.

- Tonic seizures: Tonic seizures are convulsions that involve a sudden and sustained contraction or stiffening of the muscles, typically in the arms, legs, or trunk. The person may tumble down or lose balance, and may suffer pain or discomfort. Tonic seizures normally last for a few seconds to a few minutes, and can occur during sleep or alertness. Tonic seizures are more prevalent in persons with particular forms of epilepsy, such as Lennox-Gastaut syndrome or Dravet syndrome.

- Clonic seizures: Clonic seizures are seizures that induce a fast and rhythmic contraction and relaxation of the muscles, resulting in jerking or twitching motions. The individual may lose control of their limbs, face, or torso, and may suffer difficulties breathing or speaking. Clonic seizures normally persist for a few minutes, and can occur in isolation or in conjunction with other forms of seizures. Clonic seizures are more prevalent in newborns and young children than in adults.

- Tonic-clonic seizures: Tonic-clonic seizures, commonly known as grand mal seizures, are the most severe and dramatic form of seizures. They combine the symptoms of both tonic and clonic seizures, and induce a loss of consciousness, stiffening, shaking, and convulsing of the whole body. The person may also experience biting of the tongue, frothing of the mouth, loss of bladder or bowel control, or damage. Tonic-clonic seizures normally persist for a few minutes, and can be life-threatening if not treated swiftly. Tonic-clonic seizures are the most common sort of seizures that people identify with epilepsy.

- Atonic seizures: Atonic seizures, also known as drop attacks, are seizures that produce a sudden and total loss of muscular tone or strength. The individual may collapse or fall down, and may hurt themself. Atonic seizures normally persist for a few seconds, and can occur without any warning. Atonic seizures are more prevalent in persons with particular forms of epilepsy, such as Lennox-Gastaut syndrome or Doose syndrome.

- Myoclonic seizures: Myoclonic seizures are seizures that involve quick and abrupt jerks or twitches of the muscles, commonly in the arms, legs, or upper torso. The individual may drop or fling items, or have trouble holding or controlling them. Myoclonic seizures normally endure for a fraction of a second, and can occur in clusters or in isolation. Myoclonic seizures are more prevalent in patients with particular forms of epilepsy, such as juvenile myoclonic epilepsy or progressive myoclonic epilepsy.

These are the primary types of seizures that can occur in persons with epilepsy. However, there are also other forms of seizures that are less frequent or more particular, such as gelastic seizures, epileptic spasms, or status epilepticus. These forms of seizures may require particular diagnosis and treatment, and may have varied results and implications.

Epilepsy is a complicated and diverse disorder that can have different origins, kinds, and symptoms. It is crucial to understand the nature and features of epilepsy, and to recognize the signs and symptoms of seizures. This can allow you to seek appropriate medical attention, to obtain proper diagnosis and treatment, and to prevent or limit the problems and dangers of epilepsy. It can also assist you to manage with the challenges and difficulties of living with epilepsy, and to enhance your quality of life and well-being.

CHAPTER 2

How is Epilepsy Diagnosed?

Epilepsy is a disorder that may be difficult to diagnose, since there is no one test or approach that can confirm or rule out its existence. Epilepsy is diagnosed based on a mix of criteria, such as the medical history, the physical examination, the blood tests, and the brain testing. These characteristics may assist to assess the kind, frequency, and cause of the seizures, and to rule out any other disorders that may resemble or provoke them. The diagnosis of epilepsy might take some time, since it may involve many visits, testing, and consultations. The diagnosis of epilepsy might also alter over time, as new facts, symptoms, or therapies may emerge.

The diagnosis of epilepsy is crucial, as it may assist to offer correct information, proper therapy, and enough support for the patients and their family. The diagnosis of epilepsy may also assist to avoid or lessen the consequences and hazards of epilepsy, such as injury, infection, status epilepticus, sudden unexpected death in epilepsy (SUDEP), or psychological issues. The diagnosis of epilepsy may also assist to enhance the quality of life and well-being of the patients and their families, as it can lessen the uncertainty, fear, and stigma associated with epilepsy.

In this chapter, I will discuss the many procedures and tests used to diagnose epilepsy, such as the medical history, the physical examination, the blood tests, and the brain testing. I will also describe the criteria and obstacles of diagnosing epilepsy, and how to prepare for and deal with the diagnostic process.

- Medical history: The medical history is the first and most significant stage in the diagnosis of epilepsy, as it may give useful insights and information about the seizures and their probable causes. The medical history comprises asking the patient and their family members a number of questions, such as:
 - When did the seizures start, and how frequently do they occur?
   - What are the indications and symptoms of the seizures, and how long do they last?
   - What are the triggers or things that may instigate or intensify the seizures, such as stress, lack of sleep, or flashing lights?
   - What are the results or consequences of the seizures, such as loss of consciousness, memory loss, damage, or infection?
   - How do the seizures affect the everyday lives, activities, and relationships of the patient and their family members?
   - What are the medical illnesses, drugs, allergies, or procedures that the patient or their family members have or have, particularly those that may damage the brain or the nervous system?

- What is the genetic or family history of epilepsy or seizures in the patient or their family members?

- What are the lifestyle habits or preferences of the patient, such as food, exercise, smoking, alcohol, or drugs?

The medical history may assist to determine the kind, frequency, and source of the seizures, and to rule out any other disorders that may resemble or provoke them. The medical history may also assist to select the appropriate therapy and care strategy for the patient. The medical history may be gathered via interviews, questionnaires, or forms, and it is crucial to be honest, accurate, and complete while giving it.

Physical examination: The physical examination is the second stage in the diagnosis of epilepsy, since it may serve to evaluate the overall health and function of the patient, and to discover any indications or anomalies that may signal or relate to epilepsy. The physical examination involves checking the vital signs, such as the blood pressure, the pulse, the temperature, and the respiration, and examining the various systems and organs of the body, such as the heart, the lungs, the abdomen, the skin, the eyes, the ears, the nose, the mouth, the throat, the neck, the limbs, the muscles, the joints, the reflexes, the coordination, the balance, the sensation, and the cognition. The physical examination may assist to discover any physical or mental disorders that may impact the seizures or their treatment, and to rule out any other diseases that may imitate or provoke them. The physical examination may be conducted by a general practitioner, a neurologist, or a nurse, and it is crucial to comply, follow instructions, and disclose any symptoms or concerns while undergoing it.

Blood tests: The blood tests are the third stage in the diagnosis of epilepsy, since they may assist to assess the levels and functioning of numerous chemicals and cells in the blood, and to discover any imbalances or infections that may signal or connect to epilepsy. The blood tests entail collecting a sample of blood from a vein, generally in the arm, and sending it to a laboratory for examination. The blood tests may assist to detect any metabolic, hormonal, immunological, or genetic variables that may impact the seizures or their treatment, and to rule out any other illnesses that may resemble or provoke them. The blood tests may also serve to monitor the effects or side effects of the drugs or therapies used for epilepsy. The blood tests may be requested by a general practitioner, a neurologist, or a nurse, and they are normally easy, safe, and painless, but they may cause some discomfort, bruising, or bleeding.

Brain tests: The brain tests are the fourth and last stage in the diagnosis of epilepsy, since they may help to view, record, and evaluate the structure and activity of the brain, and to determine the cause and extent of the seizures. The brain tests involve using various devices and techniques, such as the electroencephalogram (EEG), the magnetic resonance imaging (MRI), the positron emission tomography (PET), the single-photon emission computed tomography (SPECT), the computed tomography (CT), the magnetoencephalography (MEG), or the functional magnetic resonance imaging (fMRI). The brain tests may assist to confirm or reject the diagnosis of epilepsy, and to assess the kind, frequency, and source of the seizures. The brain tests may also serve to guide the therapy and management plan for the patient, and to assess the results and efficacy of the treatments. The brain tests may be conducted by a neurologist, a radiologist, or a technician, and they are normally non-invasive, safe, and painless, but they may need some preparation, cooperation, and follow-up.

These are the major procedures and tests used to diagnose epilepsy, and they may offer a thorough and trustworthy picture of the disorder and its ramifications.

Challenges And Limitations That May Affect The Diagnosis Of Epilepsy

1- The diversity and unpredictability of the seizures: The seizures may vary in frequency, length, severity, and kind, depending on the source and location of the aberrant brain activity. The seizures may sometimes occur without any warning or pattern, making them difficult to detect, document, or forecast. This may make it challenging to identify epilepsy, since it may need several or extended testing, or it may result in false negatives or false positives.

2- The similarity and overlap of the symptoms: The symptoms of the seizures might be similar or overlapping with those of other illnesses, such as migraines, fainting, panic attacks, sleep disturbances, or psychogenic non-epileptic seizures (PNES). These illnesses may imitate or provoke seizures, or they can coexist with epilepsy, making it challenging to identify epilepsy, since it may need differential or extra testing, or it may result in misdiagnosis or delayed diagnosis.

3- The lack of consciousness or recognition of the seizures: The seizures might be minor and scarcely detectable, or they can impact the awareness or memory of the individual, rendering them ignorant or oblivious of what is occurring during or after the seizure. The seizures might also be misinterpreted or disregarded by the individual or their family members, making them unwilling or unable to seek medical assistance or offer correct information. This may make it challenging to identify epilepsy, since it may lead to underreporting or underestimate of the seizures, or it may result in denial or stigma.

Standards and problems of diagnosing epilepsy

Epilepsy is a disorder that affects the brain and produces frequent seizures. Seizures are rapid bursts of electrical activity in the brain that may influence how a person feels or acts. Epilepsy may have many diverse causes, such as brain damage, infection, stroke, hereditary factors, or unexplained reasons. Diagnosing epilepsy may be tricky, since not all seizures are apparent and there is no one test that can prove the disease. Here are some criteria and obstacles of diagnosing epilepsy, and how to prepare for and deal with the diagnostic process.

Criteria for diagnosing epilepsy: According to the International League Against Epilepsy (ILAE), the criteria for diagnosing epilepsy are:

-Having at least two unprovoked (or reflex) seizures occurring more than 24 hours apart.
   *Having one unprovoked (or reflex) seizure and a chance of subsequent seizures comparable to the overall recurrence risk (at least 60%) after two unprovoked seizures, happening during the following 10 years.
*Having a diagnosis of epileptic syndrome.

Challenges of diagnosing epilepsy

Some of the complications of diagnosing epilepsy are:

1- Seizures may have varied forms, causes, and triggers, and they can vary in frequency, length, and severity. Some seizures may not create any obvious symptoms, while others may be mistaken for other ailments, such as fainting, migraines, or sleep disorders.

2- There is no conclusive test for epilepsy. The diagnosis is based on a mix of medical history, physical and neurological examination, blood tests, and brain imaging and recording methods, such as electroencephalogram (EEG), computed tomography (CT) scan, magnetic resonance imaging (MRI), or functional MRI (fMRI). However, these tests may not always provide unambiguous evidence of epilepsy or its etiology, and they may have limits, hazards, or costs.

3- The diagnosis may take time and need many visits to various experts, such as neurologists, epileptologists, psychiatrists, psychologists, or geneticists. The diagnosis may also alter over time, as new information or test findings become available, or as the seizures develop or react to therapy.

How to prepare for the diagnostic process:

Some of the methods to prepare for the diagnosis process are:

1- Keep a seizure journal, where you write the date, time, length, type, and probable triggers of each seizure, as well as how you felt before, during, and after the seizure. You may also use a smartphone app or a wearable gadget to monitor your seizures.

2- Bring a family member, friend, or caregiver who saw your seizures to your visits. They may give crucial information about what occurred, particularly if you were unconscious or disoriented during the seizure.

3-Write down any questions or concerns you have regarding your disease, symptoms, testing, or treatment choices. You may also bring a list of your current drugs, allergies, and medical issues.

4- Be honest and transparent with your healthcare staff. Tell them about any changes in your seizures, mood, memory, or behavior. Ask them to clarify anything you do not understand, and get a second opinion if you are not pleased with the diagnosis or treatment plan.

How to deal with the diagnostic process:
Some of the strategies to deal with the diagnostic process are:

1-Seek assistance from your family, friends, or caretakers. They may assist you with practical activities, such as driving, cooking, or shopping, as well as emotional support, such as listening, soothing, or encouraging you.

2- Join a support group, online network, or advocacy organization for persons with epilepsy or seizures. You may share your experiences, learn from others, and uncover tools and information that can help you manage your illness.

3- Educate yourself about epilepsy and seizures. Learn about the numerous forms, causes, and treatments of epilepsy, and how to avoid or react to seizures. You may also find out about your rights and duties as a person with epilepsy, such as driving, working, or traveling.

4- Take care of your physical and mental wellness. Follow your treatment plan, take your medicines as directed, and avoid any triggers or risk factors that may increase your seizures. You may also adopt a healthy lifestyle, such as eating properly, sleeping sufficiently, exercising frequently, and decreasing stress. If you have any indications of depression, anxiety, or other mental health difficulties, get professional treatment as soon as possible.

CHAPTER 3

Exploring the Treatment Options for Epilepsy:

Epilepsy is a neurological illness that produces repeated seizures, which are rapid and abnormal bursts of electrical activity in the brain. There are several approaches to treat epilepsy, depending on the kind, frequency, and severity of the seizures, as well as the patient's age, medical history, and preferences. Some of the most prevalent treatment options are:

- Medication:
Anti-seizure medications, often known as anticonvulsants or antiepileptic drugs, are the basis of epilepsy therapy. They act by lowering the excitability of the brain cells that produce seizures. There are many distinct types of anti-seizure medications, each with its unique mechanism of action, efficacy, and adverse effects. Some of the most extensively used anti-seizure medications include carbamazepine, valproate, phenytoin, lamotrigine, levetiracetam, and topiramate. The choice of medicine relies on various aspects, such as the kind of seizures, the patient's age, gender, weight, liver and kidney function, and other drugs they are taking. The amount and frequency of medicine may also vary from person to person, and may need to be changed over time. The objective of medicine is to

provide seizure control with the lowest feasible dosage and the fewest adverse effects. Some of the typical adverse effects of anti-seizure medicines include sleepiness, dizziness, nausea, rash, weight gain or loss, and mood changes. Some anti-seizure medicines may potentially interact with other drugs, such as birth control pills, antibiotics, and blood thinners, and impair their efficacy or induce unpleasant responses. Therefore, it is vital to visit a doctor before beginning, stopping, or modifying any medicine, and to notify them of any additional medications or supplements the patient is taking. It is also vital to take the drug as recommended, and not to miss or skip doses, since this may raise the risk of seizures or withdrawal symptoms.

- Surgery:
Surgery is a possibility for certain patients with epilepsy who have focal seizures, which are seizures that originate in a particular portion of the brain. Surgery includes removing or disconnecting the section of the brain that is producing the seizures, generally a tiny region in the temporal or frontal lobe. operation may be considered when the seizures are not controlled by medication, when the seizure focus can be clearly defined and localized, and when the operation will not cause major impairment to the brain functions, such as memory, language, or mobility. Surgery may be able to decrease or eliminate the seizures, or at least make them less frequent or severe. However, surgery also entails certain dangers, such as infection, hemorrhage, stroke, or neurological damage. Therefore, surgery is

only recommended after a thorough evaluation by a team of specialists, including neurologists, neurosurgeons, neuropsychologists, and epileptologists, who will assess the benefits and risks of the procedure, and explain the possible outcomes and expectations to the patient and their family. Surgery is generally followed by a period of recuperation and rehabilitation, and may need continuing usage of medication to prevent or treat any lingering or new seizures.

- Vagus Nerve Stimulation (VNS): VNS is a form of neuromodulation, which is a treatment that employs electrical stimulation to affect the activity of the nervous system. VNS includes implanting a tiny device beneath the skin of the chest, which is attached to a wire that wraps around the vagus nerve in the neck. The vagus nerve is a key nerve that links the brain to numerous organs, such as the heart, lungs, and stomach. The gadget sends modest pulses of electricity to the vagus nerve at regular intervals, generally every few minutes. The stimulation is believed to influence the brain circuits that are involved in seizures, and to lower the frequency and severity of seizures. VNS may be an alternative for persons with epilepsy who have partial or generalized seizures that are not adequately managed by medication, and who are not ideal candidates for surgery. VNS may also have some favorable impacts on mood, memory, and quality of life. However, VNS also has several limits and adverse effects, such as the requirement for surgery to implant and replace the device, the chance of device failure or infection, and the incidence of side symptoms such as hoarseness, cough, shortness of breath, or tingling in the neck during stimulation. Therefore, VNS involves careful identification of applicants, modification of stimulation settings, and continuous monitoring by a clinician.

- Responsive Neurostimulation (RNS):
RNS is another kind of neuromodulation, which is similar to VNS, except instead of stimulating the vagus nerve, it stimulates the brain directly. RNS includes implanting a tiny device in the skull, which is coupled to one or two wires that are put into the brain, near the location where the seizures originate. The equipment analyzes the brain activity and identifies any odd patterns that may suggest an oncoming seizure. When it recognizes such a pattern, it provides a burst of electrical stimulation to the brain, to halt the seizure before it spreads. RNS may be a choice for persons with epilepsy who have focal seizures that are not managed by medication or surgery, and who have one or two well-defined seizure foci. RNS may be able to lessen the frequency and severity of seizures, and may help enhance cognitive and emotional functioning. However, RNS also has certain negatives and dangers, such as the requirement for surgery to implant and replace the device, the likelihood of device failure or infection, and the development of side effects such as headache, discomfort, or infection at the implant site. Therefore, RNS involves careful screening of applicants, modification of stimulation levels, and continuous follow-up by a specialist.

- Ketogenic Diet:

Ketogenic diet is a unique diet that is rich in fat, low in carbohydrate, and sufficient in protein. It is meant to replicate the metabolic state of hunger, in which the body utilizes fat instead of glucose as its major source of energy. This leads in the formation of ketone bodies, which are molecules that may penetrate the blood-brain barrier and offer an alternate fuel for the brain. The ketogenic diet is hypothesized to have an anticonvulsant impact, by modifying the balance of neurotransmitters, lowering inflammation, and boosting the function of mitochondria, the energy-producing components of the cells. The ketogenic diet may be an option for persons with epilepsy who have drug-resistant seizures, particularly children with specific disorders, such as Lennox-Gastaut syndrome, Dravet syndrome, or tuberous sclerosis. The ketogenic diet may be able to lessen the frequency and severity of seizures, and may also enhance cognitive and behavioral results. However, the ketogenic diet also has certain problems and side effects, such as the difficulty of following the diet, the necessity for constant monitoring by a nutritionist and a doctor, and the incidence of side effects such as constipation, dehydration, kidney stones, growth retardation, or bone loss. Therefore, the ketogenic diet demands careful identification of candidates, computation of the food composition, and frequent monitoring of the blood levels of ketones, glucose, and electrolytes.

- Cannabidiol (CBD):

CBD is a chemical that is derived from the cannabis plant, which is also known as marijuana. CBD is one of the numerous cannabinoids, which are substances that operate on the cannabinoid receptors in the brain and other regions of the body. CBD is distinct from tetrahydrocannabinol (THC), which is the major psychoactive component of cannabis that creates the "high" experience. CBD does not have any psychotropic effects, but it may have some anticonvulsant effects, via altering the activity of many neurotransmitter systems, such as glutamate, GABA, serotonin, and adenosine. CBD may be a possibility for persons with epilepsy who suffer seizures that are resistant to standard therapies, particularly children with unusual and severe types of epilepsy, such as Dravet syndrome or Lennox-Gastaut syndrome. CBD may be able to lower the frequency and severity of seizures, and may also enhance the quality of life and sleep. However, CBD also has several limits and adverse effects, such as the absence of standardized and controlled products, the likelihood of medicine interactions or contamination, and the incidence of side effects such as diarrhea, lethargy, appetite loss, or liver issues. Therefore, CBD needs careful screening of applicants, calculation of the best dosage and formulation, and frequent review by a specialist.

These are some of the numerous choices and tactics for treating epilepsy. Each of them has its own pros and downsides, and none of them is a perfect or guaranteed answer. The optimum therapy for each person with epilepsy relies on their specific condition and requirements, and may entail a mix of various techniques. The therapy should be personalized to the patient's objectives and preferences, and should be evaluated and altered frequently, depending on the reaction and feedback. The therapy should also be accompanied by additional measures, including as education, counseling, lifestyle modifications, and seizure management plans, to increase the efficacy and safety of the treatment, and to improve the overall well-being and quality of life of the person with epilepsy and their family.

First aid for epilepsy seizures

Epilepsy is a disorder that affects the brain and produces frequent seizures. Seizures are rapid bursts of electrical activity in the brain that may influence how a person feels or behaves. Some seizures might cause a person to lose consciousness, collapse, tremble, or become disoriented. Seizures may be alarming, but most of them are not emergencies and can be controlled with easy actions. Here are some basic ideas on how to support someone who is suffering a seizure:

1- remain calm and remain with the individual until the seizure is ended. Most seizures last just a few minutes and end by themselves.

2- Keep the individual safe by taking away anything that might damage them, such as sharp or hot materials. If the individual is roaming or in a risky situation, gently lead them to a safer position.

3- Make the individual comfortable by helping them sit or lay down. If they are laying down, flip them on their side to assist them breathe. Put something soft beneath their head, such as a jacket or a cushion. Loosen any tight clothing around their neck, such as a tie or a scarf.

4- Do not hold the individual down or attempt to halt their movements. This may cause greater damage or injury. Let the seizure take its course.

5- Do not put anything in the person's mouth, such as a spoon, a finger, or a wallet. This may injure their teeth, jaw, or tongue. It may also restrict their airway and make it difficult to breathe. Contrary to a frequent belief, a person cannot swallow their tongue during a seizure.

6- Do not offer the individual anything to drink or eat until they are completely awake and aware. They may choke or aspirate on the food or drink.

7- Check the person's respiration and pulse following the seizure. If they are not breathing or have no pulse, call for immediate aid and start CPR if you know how.

8- Time the seizure and record what occurred. This might assist the client and their doctor understand their situation better. Write down how long the seizure lasted, what sort of seizure it was, and what symptoms the individual experienced before, during, and after the seizure.

9- Call for emergency aid if the seizure lasts more than 5 minutes, or if the individual has another seizure shortly after the first one. Also contact for aid if the individual is wounded, pregnant, diabetic, or has a heart disease. If the individual has never had a seizure before, or does not have a diagnosis of epilepsy, they should consult a doctor as soon as possible.

10- Be helpful and comforting to the individual following the seizure. They may feel puzzled, fatigued, or ashamed. Tell them what occurred and where they are. Help them rest or go home securely. Do not leave them alone till they have completely healed.

CHAPTER 4

How to maintain a healthy lifestyle with epilepsy

A healthy lifestyle is crucial for everyone, but particularly for persons with epilepsy. A healthy lifestyle may help decrease the frequency and severity of seizures, boost mood and energy levels, and prevent or manage other health issues.

Some of the main parts of a healthy lifestyle are:

1- Eating a balanced diet that contains lots of fruits, vegetables, whole grains, lean protein, and healthy fats. Avoiding items that may provoke seizures, such as coffee, alcohol, artificial sweeteners, and processed foods .

2- Getting adequate sleep and rest. Lack of sleep may raise the risk of seizures and impact mental and physical health. Aim for at least seven to eight hours of sleep every night and adopt a regular sleep routine .

3- Exercising consistently and safely. Exercise may improve cardiovascular health, build muscles and bones, decrease stress, and promote mood and self-esteem. Choose activities that are pleasant and suitable for your fitness level and seizure type. Avoid activities that may provide a danger of injury or drowning, such as swimming, climbing, or riding alone .

4- Taking drugs as recommended and following the doctor's advice. Medications are the primary therapy for epilepsy and may help control seizures and avoid problems. It is vital to take drugs precisely as recommended, without skipping doses or modifying the dosage. It is also vital to advise the doctor of any negative effects, allergies, or interactions with other medicines or supplements .

5- Keeping a seizure journal and monitoring your triggers. A seizure diary is a record of when, when, and how seizures occur, as well as any variables that may have contributed to them, such as stress, sickness, menstruation, or prescription changes. A seizure journal may assist in detecting patterns and causes of seizures, assess the success of therapy, and give helpful information for the clinician and the patient .

Sudden unexplained death in epilepsy (SUDEP)

Sudden unexplained death in epilepsy (SUDEP) is an uncommon but significant complication of epilepsy that happens when a person with epilepsy dies abruptly and no other cause of death can be determined. The specific cause of SUDEP is not understood, although some suspected variables are:

- Breathing issues: A seizure may cause a person to cease breathing (apnea) or have trouble breathing (dyspnea), which may deplete the oxygen level in the blood and lead to brain damage or cardiac arrest. A seizure may also cause a person's airway to become choked or restricted, resulting in asphyxia.

- **Heart issues:** A seizure may produce a change in the heart rhythm (arrhythmia) or the heart rate (tachycardia or bradycardia), which may disrupt the blood supply to the brain and other organs. A seizure may potentially cause the heart to cease beating (cardiac arrest) or to beat excessively fast or too slow (cardiac dysrhythmia).

- **Other or combined causes:** SUDEP may develop from a combination of respiratory and cardiac issues, or from other unknown variables that impact the brain or the body during or after a seizure.

Some risk factors that may enhance the chance of SUDEP are:

- Having frequent or uncontrollable seizures, particularly generalized tonic-clonic seizures (also known as grand mal seizures) that impact the entire brain and body.
- Having seizures at night or during sleeping, which may go undiagnosed or untreated.
- Having a lengthy duration of epilepsy or an early age of onset.
- Having additional medical disorders or illnesses that impact the brain, the heart, or the lungs.
- Taking various anti-seizure drugs or changing medications often.
- Not taking anti-seizure drugs as recommended or skipping doses.
- Drinking alcohol or taking recreational drugs.

SUDEP is not very prevalent, but it is vital to be aware of the danger and take precautions to avoid it. Some suggested approaches to lower the risk of SUDEP are:

- Taking anti-seizure meds as indicated and following up with the doctor frequently.
- Avoiding factors that may induce seizures, such as stress, sleep deprivation, flashing lights, or specific meals.
- Having a seizure action plan and alerting family, friends, and caregivers on what to do in case of a seizure.
- Using a seizure warning device or a monitoring system that can identify seizures and notify someone for aid.
- Sleeping on the side or using a pillow that may avoid suffocation.
- Seeking medical care if seizures vary in frequency, severity, or length.

How to manage stress, anxiety, and depression with epilepsy?

Stress, anxiety, and sadness are frequent emotional issues for persons with epilepsy. They may impact the quality of life, the capacity to live with epilepsy, and the risk of seizures.

Some of the strategies to manage with stress, anxiety, and depression are:

- **Seeking professional aid:** A mental health practitioner, such as a psychologist, psychiatrist, or counselor, may offer diagnosis, treatment, and support for mental health disorders. They may provide numerous treatments, such as cognitive-behavioral therapy, interpersonal therapy, or mindfulness-based therapy, that can help transform negative attitudes and behaviors, increase coping abilities, and boost well-being .

- **Joining a support group:** A support group is a collection of individuals who share similar experiences and problems, such as living with epilepsy. A support group may give emotional support, practical assistance, and a feeling of belonging and community. Support groups may be accessed online or offline, via local organizations, hospitals, or websites .

- **Practicing relaxing methods:** Relaxation techniques are strategies that may help relieve stress, anxiety, and depression by soothing the body and the mind. Some examples of relaxation methods include deep breathing, gradual muscle relaxation, meditation, yoga, tai chi, or music therapy .

- **Engaging in pleasurable and meaningful activities:** Activities that offer delight and satisfaction may assist increase mood, self-esteem, and motivation. They may also distract from bad feelings and create a sense of purpose and success. Some examples of fun and meaningful activities include hobbies, volunteering, learning, or spending time with friends and family .

Memory and cognition are mental processes that entail thinking, learning, remembering, and problem-solving. Epilepsy may influence memory and cognition in numerous ways, such as producing memory loss, disorientation, trouble focusing, or sluggish processing speed.

Some of the strategies to increase memory and cognition are:

- **Stimulating the brain:** The brain is like a muscle that requires exercise to be healthy and sharp. Brain stimulation may assist enhance memory and cognition by improving brain connections, boosting blood flow, and delaying cognitive decline. Some forms of brain stimulation include puzzles, gaming, reading, writing, or acquiring new abilities .

- **Organizing and simplifying information:** Information that is structured and simplified is simpler to recall and comprehend. Organizing and simplifying information may assist enhance memory and cognition by minimizing mental clutter, boosting attention, and strengthening recall. Some ways of organizing and simplifying information include generating lists, utilizing calendars, setting reminders, employing mnemonics, or chunking information .

- Repeating and reviewing information: Information that is repeated and reviewed is more likely to be preserved and retrieved in the long-term memory. Repeating and revisiting material may assist enhance memory and cognition by strengthening memory traces, consolidating learning, and boosting retrieval. Some instances of repeating and reviewing material include rehearsing, summarizing, testing, or instructing .

- Seeking feedback and direction: Feedback and guidance are kinds of external input that may assist enhance memory and cognition by giving correction, explanation, or reinforcement. Feedback and advice may come from numerous sources, such as instructors, tutors, coaches, mentors, or peers .

How to boost self-esteem and confidence with epilepsy?

Self-esteem and confidence are sentiments of self-worth and self-efficacy that reflect how one regards oneself and one's talents. Epilepsy may impair self-esteem and confidence in numerous ways, such as producing negative self-image, self-doubt, or social isolation. Some of the strategies to boost self-esteem and confidence are:

- Challenging negative self-talk: Negative self-talk is the inner voice that criticizes, judges, or blames oneself. Negative self-talk may impair self-esteem and confidence by producing a skewed and inaccurate self-image. Challenging negative self-talk may help boost self-esteem and confidence by replacing negative beliefs with positive or realistic ones .

- **Setting and attaining goals:** Goals are desirable outcomes that one desires to reach. Goals may enhance self-esteem and confidence by offering direction, motivation, and feedback. Setting and attaining objectives may help increase self-esteem and confidence by generating a feeling of purpose, progress, and success .

- **Celebrating strengths and triumphs:** Strengths and successes are positive traits and results that one has or accomplishes. Strengths and triumphs may enhance self-esteem and confidence by recognizing one's talents and accomplishments. Celebrating strengths and triumphs may help increase self-esteem and confidence by identifying, praising, and awarding oneself .

- **Seeking and receiving support:** Support is the aid and encouragement that one gets from others. Support may boost self-esteem and confidence by offering emotional, practical, or informational aid. Seeking and receiving assistance may help build self-esteem and confidence by recognizing, trusting, and appreciating oneself and others .

Education, job, and hobbies are significant areas of life that entail learning, working, and having pleasure. Epilepsy may influence education, job, and hobbies in numerous ways, such as providing academic difficulty, work obstacles, or activity constraints.
Some of the methods to pursue education, profession, and interests are:
- **Exploring options and possibilities:** Options and opportunities are the choices and chances that one has or may generate in life. Options and chances may assist pursue education, job, and hobbies by increasing one's horizons, interests, and ambitions. Exploring possibilities and chances may assist pursue education, profession, and hobbies by studying, networking, or trying .
- **Planning and preparing:** Planning and preparing are the activities of developing and organizing the procedures and resources required to accomplish a desired goal. Planning and planning may assist pursue education, job, and hobbies by boosting one's efficiency, effectiveness, and preparedness. Planning and preparation may assist pursue education, job, and hobbies by creating targets, plans, and contingencies .
- **Adapting and adjusting:** Adapting and adjusting are the capacities to alter and deal with changes or problems in life. Adapting and modifying may assist in pursuing education, job, and hobbies by strengthening one's flexibility, resilience, and problem-solving abilities.

Adapting and adapting may assist pursue education, job, and hobbies by altering expectations, techniques, or activities .

   - Advocating and asserting: Advocating and asserting are the abilities of speaking out and standing up for oneself and one's rights. Advocating and asserting may assist pursue education, profession, and hobbies by safeguarding one's interests, needs, and preferences. Advocating and asserting may assist pursue education, profession, and hobbies by talking, bargaining, or seeking .

CHAPTER 5

Epilepsy in children

Epilepsy in children is a disorder that affects the brain and produces seizures. A seizure is a quick burst of aberrant electrical activity in the brain that may alter how a kid feels, thinks, or moves. Seizures may have varied symptoms and linger for varying durations of time. Some seizures may cause a kid to lose consciousness, while others may merely produce a momentary shift in awareness or behavior.

There are several varieties of epilepsy in children, and each one has its own features and causes. Some of the most frequent kinds are:

- **Absence epilepsy:** This form involves short bouts of staring and unresponsiveness, generally lasting less than 10 seconds. A youngster may experience hundreds of these seizures a day, which may interfere with learning and concentration. Absence epilepsy normally develops between ages 4 and 12 and frequently goes away by adolescence.
- **Rolandic epilepsy:** This kind involves seizures that affect the face, tongue, or neck, generally on one side of the body. A youngster may suffer twitching, tingling, or numbness in these regions, or have problems speaking

or swallowing. Rolandic epilepsy commonly happens at night, when a kid is falling asleep or waking up. It commonly begins between years 3 and 13 and usually fades away by age 16.

- **Juvenile myoclonic epilepsy:** This kind involves seizures that include abrupt jerking movements of the arms, legs, or upper torso. A youngster may drop or hurl stuff, or tumble down. Juvenile myoclonic epilepsy normally begins around puberty and frequently persists throughout adulthood. It is generally induced by lack of sleep, stress, or alcohol.

- **Infantile spasms:** This kind involves seizures that include short, recurrent spasms of the muscles, notably in the neck, back, and arms. A youngster may bend forward, arch backward, or curl up. Infantile spasms frequently occur in clusters, many times a day, and are more likely when a kid is falling asleep or waking up. They often start between ages 3 and 12 months and may cause developmental delays or regression[1].

- **Lennox-Gastaut syndrome:** This variety includes many types of seizures, including tonic (stiffening), atonic (dropping), and absence (staring) seizures. A youngster may experience frequent falls, bruises, or loss of consciousness. Lennox-Gastaut syndrome normally develops between ages 2 and 6 and frequently continues into adulthood. It is commonly connected with brain abnormalities or traumas.

The causes of epilepsy in children are not usually understood, although some likely reasons include:

- **Genetic factors:** Some kinds of epilepsy in children are inherited or run in families. Other kinds are caused by mutations or alterations in the genes that impact brain development or function.
- **Brain disorders:** Some kinds of epilepsy in children are caused by abnormalities or injuries in the brain, such as tumors, strokes, infections, deformities, or trauma. These may disrupt how the brain cells interact with one other and produce seizures.
- **Metabolic or immunological disorders:** Some kinds of epilepsy in children are caused by difficulties with the body's metabolism or immune system, such as low blood sugar, electrolyte imbalance, autoimmune illnesses, or inflammation. These may impair the brain's function and induce seizures.
- **Unknown factors:** In certain situations, the etiology of epilepsy in children is unknown or idiopathic. This indicates that there is no apparent rationale for why the seizures occur.

Diagnosis of epilepsy in children

The diagnosis of epilepsy in children is based on the child's medical history, physical examination, and testing. Some of the tests that may be utilized are:

- **Electroencephalogram (EEG):** This test monitors the electrical activity of the brain using electrodes connected to the scalp. It may indicate the location and kind of seizures, as well as the pattern and frequency of the brain waves.
- **Magnetic resonance imaging (MRI):** This test employs a strong magnetic field and radio waves to obtain detailed pictures of the brain. It may reveal the structure and architecture of the brain, as well as any anomalies or lesions that may trigger seizures.
- **Blood testing:** These tests may screen for the levels of glucose, electrolytes, hormones, and other chemicals in the blood that may impact the brain's function and trigger seizures.
- **Genetic testing:** These tests may examine the existence of certain genes or mutations that may cause or increase the risk of seizures.

Treatment of epilepsy in children

The treatment of epilepsy in children varies on the kind and intensity of the seizures, as well as the child's age, health, and preferences. Some of the therapeutic possibilities are:

- **Medications:** These are medications that help decrease or prevent seizures by changing the brain's chemical balance or electrical activity. There are several sorts of drugs for epilepsy, and each one has its own advantages and negative effects. A youngster may need to try several drugs or combinations of medications to discover the most effective and comfortable one.

- **Surgery:** This is a technique that eliminates or disconnects the portion of the brain that causes seizures. It is typically considered when drugs are not helpful or create unbearable side effects, and when the seizures are confined to a particular location of the brain that may be safely operated on. Surgery may lessen or eliminate seizures in certain circumstances, but it may potentially have dangers or problems.
- **Dietary therapy:** This is a specific diet that adjusts the quantity or type of carbs, lipids, and proteins that a youngster consumes. It may modify the brain's metabolism and prevent seizures in certain circumstances. The most popular dietary treatment for epilepsy is the ketogenic diet, which is rich in fat and low in carbs. Other dietary treatments include the modified Atkins diet, the low glycemic index therapy, and the medium chain triglyceride diet.

- **Vagus nerve stimulation (VNS):** This is a device that provides electrical impulses to the vagus nerve, which is a major nerve that links the brain to the body. It may help lower the frequency and severity of seizures in certain individuals. The device is implanted beneath the skin of the chest and attached to a cable that wraps around the vagus nerve in the neck. The gadget may be set to send shocks at regular intervals or when actuated by a magnet.

- **Responsive neurostimulation (RNS):** This is a device that detects and reacts to the brain's electrical activity. It may help identify and stop seizures before they spread or become obvious. The device is implanted in the skull and attached to electrodes that are put in or near the region of the brain that produces seizures. The gadget can recognize aberrant electrical impulses and apply stimulation to stop them.

- **Deep brain stimulation (DBS):** This is a device that sends electrical impulses to particular areas in the brain. It may assist control the brain's activity and minimize seizures in certain circumstances. The gadget is implanted in the chest and linked to wires that are put into the brain via tiny holes in the skull. The gadget may be set to send impulses at varying frequencies or intensities.

Challenges encountered by children with Epilepsy

Epilepsy in children may influence their quality of life, growth, and learning. Some of the obstacles that children with epilepsy may experience are:

- **Seizure-related injuries or accidents:** Children with epilepsy may suffer falls, burns, bites, or bruises during or after a seizure. They may also have trouble breathing, swallowing, or speaking. They may require medical treatment or emergency care in certain circumstances.

- **adverse effects of drugs or therapies:** Children with epilepsy may encounter adverse effects from the medications or treatments that they take or receive. These may include sleepiness, dizziness, nausea, vomiting, weight gain, mood changes, cognitive issues, or allergic reactions. They may need to change their dosage or switch to new drugs or therapies in certain circumstances.

- **Social and emotional issues:** Children with epilepsy may feel different, alienated, or ostracized by their classmates, teachers, or others. They may have poor self-esteem, anxiety, sadness, or behavioral difficulties. They may require therapy, support groups, or other assistance to deal with their emotions and problems.

- **Learning and cognitive difficulties:** Children with epilepsy may have issues with attention, concentration, memory, language, or logic. They may have inferior academic performance, school attendance, or graduation rates. They may require special schooling, accommodations, or interventions to help them learn and achieve.

Epilepsy in children is a chronic illness that needs continuing care and treatment. However, many children with epilepsy may have normal and meaningful lives with correct medication and care. Some children may outgrow their epilepsy or have fewer or no seizures as they grow older. Some children may attain seizure independence or remission with drugs or therapy. Some youngsters may learn to manage their epilepsy and conquer their problems. Epilepsy in children is not a barrier to reaching their goals and objectives

Epilepsy in adolescent

Adolescence is a time of life that comprises various physical, psychological, and social changes. It is a period when young people build their personality, freedom, and relationships. Adolescence may be tough for anybody, but particularly for those who suffer epilepsy. Epilepsy may influence several parts of a young person's life, such as:

- **Self-image and self-esteem:** Adolescence is a period of heightened self-consciousness, with exaggerated worries about physical and social appearance. Having epilepsy may make a young person feel strange, alienated, or ostracized. They may worry about how others see them, or how their seizures may effect their future. They may also encounter adverse effects from their medicine, such as weight gain, acne, or mood changes, that may impact their look and confidence.

- **Education and learning:** Epilepsy may influence a young person's academic performance and accomplishment. Seizures may affect learning and memory, and induce absences from school. Medication may also impact focus, attention, and motivation. Some young people may require special help or accommodations at school, such as more time for examinations, a quiet space to relax, or a seizure response plan. They may also require help and counseling to prepare for their job and additional education.

- **Social and emotional development:** Epilepsy may influence a young person's social and emotional well-being. They may feel lonely, sad, nervous, or resentful about their situation. They may endure bullying, prejudice, or exclusion from their peers. They may also have challenges in building and sustaining friendships and love relationships. They may need to manage with the stress of managing their epilepsy, such as taking medicine, avoiding triggers, and coping with the unpredictability of seizures. They may also need to combine their desire for independence and autonomy with their need for safety and assistance.

- **Lifestyle and activities:** Epilepsy may influence a young person's lifestyle and activities. They may have to restrict or avoid some items that might raise their risk of seizures, such as alcohol, drugs, sleep deprivation, or flashing lights. They may also experience limits or obstacles in acquiring a driver's license, traveling, or engaging in sports and hobbies. They may need to alter their lifestyle and activities to accommodate their epilepsy, and discover methods to enjoy themselves without jeopardizing their health.

Epilepsy in adolescence may be tough to live with, but it can also be controlled and cured. There are various sources of aid and support available for young people with epilepsy and their families, such as:

- **Medical professionals:** A young person with epilepsy should have frequent check-ups with their doctor or neurologist, who can monitor their condition, give medication, and refer them to other experts if required. They may also give information and guidance on different areas of epilepsy, such as diagnosis, therapy, seizure kinds, and epileptic syndromes.
- **Epilepsy nurses:** An epilepsy nurse is a nurse who specializes in epilepsy care. They may give information, counseling, and support to young individuals with epilepsy and their families. They may also aid with medication management, seizure monitoring, and emergency care.
- **Epilepsy organizations:** There are several epilepsy organizations that provide different services and

resources for young people with epilepsy and their families, such as helplines, websites, newsletters, publications, support groups, events, and advocacy. Some examples of epilepsy organizations include [Epilepsy Society] [Epilepsy Foundation] and [NICE]
- **epileptic communities:** There are several epileptic communities that give chances for young people with epilepsy and their families to interact, share, and learn from one another. They may also give emotional and social support, and improve awareness and understanding of epilepsy. Some examples of epilepsy communities include online forums, blogs, podcasts, social media, and peer networks.

Epilepsy in adolescence is a complicated and hard illness, but it is not a barrier to having a meaningful and successful life. With the correct therapy, support, and attitude, young individuals with epilepsy may overcome their problems and accomplish their objectives. They may also contribute to the epilepsy community and society, and inspire others with their tales and experiences..

Education for children and adolescents suffering epilepsy

Epilepsy may have different causes, such as hereditary factors, brain damage, infection, or stroke. Epilepsy may also influence a person's learning, memory, temperament, and social skills.

Children and adolescents with epilepsy may confront several problems in their schooling, such as:

1- Missing school days or courses due to seizures, medical visits, or adverse effects of medication.
2- Having difficulty with focus, attention, memory, or processing information, which might influence their academic achievement and self-esteem.
3- Experiencing stigma, prejudice, bullying, or isolation from their friends or teachers, who may not understand epilepsy or how to aid them during or after a seizure.
4- Being excluded from various activities, such as sports, camps, or field trips, owing to safety concerns or lack of support.
5- Having special educational needs or disabilities (SEND) that need extra help or changes in the school setting.

However, with adequate care and assistance, children and adolescents with epilepsy may have a good and successful school experience. Some of the techniques to do this are:

1- Having a personalized epilepsy management plan that covers the kind and frequency of seizures, the triggers and warning signs, the first aid and post-seizure care, the prescription and emergency medicine, and the contact information of the parents and the doctor. This plan should be shared with the school personnel, notably the teachers, the school nurse, and the bus driver, and updated periodically.

2- Having an individualized education plan (IEP) or a 504 plan that describes the academic objectives, the accommodations, the adjustments, and the assistance that the child or teenager requires to access the curriculum and engage in school activities. This plan should be established in consultation with the parents, the instructors, the school counselor, and the special education coordinator, and revised frequently.

3- Educating the school community about epilepsy and seizures, and eliminating any misunderstandings or preconceptions. This may be done by offering information and resources, such as books, posters, fact sheets, or films, to the school personnel and the kids. The Epilepsy Foundation and the Epilepsy Society provide numerous education programs and resources that might assist improve awareness and knowledge of epilepsy in schools.

4- Encouraging the child or teenager to be active in their own education and epilepsy care, and to express their wants and preferences to their parents and instructors. This may help children build self-confidence, self-advocacy, and independent skills.

5- Providing emotional and social support to the child or teenager, and helping them deal with any problems or difficulties they may experience. This may be done by listening to their thoughts and worries, complimenting their efforts and successes, encouraging their talents and interests, and connecting them with other peers or mentors who have epilepsy or comparable experiences.

By working together, parents, teachers, and health professionals can provide a safe and inclusive educational environment for children and adolescents with epilepsy, and help them attain their full potential..

Social life:
Children and adolescents living with epilepsy may confront various obstacles in their social life, such as stigma, discrimination, bullying, isolation, or exclusion from particular activities. These obstacles might influence their self-esteem, confidence, and feeling of belonging. However, with correct education, awareness, and support, children and adolescents living with epilepsy may have healthy and meaningful social interactions with their classmates, teachers, and others. They may also join in numerous social activities, such as clubs, hobbies, sports, camps, or field excursions, that fit their interests and talents. Some of the approaches to enhance social engagement and involvement for children and adolescents living with epilepsy are:

1- Educate the school and the community about epilepsy and seizures, and eliminate any misunderstandings or misconceptions.
2- Encouraging the kid or teenager to be open and honest about their epilepsy, and to seek care when required.
3- Providing emotional and social support to the child or teenager, and helping them deal with any problems or difficulties they may experience.

4- Connecting the child or teenager with other peers or mentors who have epilepsy or comparable experiences, such as via support groups, online forums, or camps.
5- Finding and accessing suitable programs and services that provide adapted or therapeutic sports and leisure for children and adolescents with disabilities.

Family life:
 Children and adolescents living with epilepsy may also have an affect on their family life, such as their parents, siblings, and other relatives. Epilepsy may bring stress, concern, anxiety, or guilt for the family members, who may have to deal with the uncertainty, unpredictability, and repercussions of seizures. Epilepsy may also impair the family's everyday routines, money, ambitions, and objectives. However, with correct knowledge, advice, and support, families of children and adolescents living with epilepsy may have a good and healthy family life. They may also offer a supporting and loving atmosphere for the kid or teenager, and assist them fulfill their potential. Some of the strategies to increase family well-being and functioning for children and adolescents living with epilepsy are:

1- Seeking and receiving correct and up-to-date information regarding epilepsy and its care, and sharing it with the family members.
2- Communicating and coordinating with the health care providers, the school staff, and other professionals engaged in the child or adolescent's care.

3- Seeking and gaining emotional and practical assistance from the family, friends, or other sources, such as counselors, social workers, or support groups.
4- Balancing the demands and obligations of the child or teenager with epilepsy and the other family members, and ensuring a healthy lifestyle for the entire family.
5- Celebrating the successes and qualities of the child or teenager with epilepsy and the other family members, and spending quality time together.

Physical life:
 Children and adolescents living with epilepsy may also have certain challenges in their physical lives, such as their health, fitness, and safety. Epilepsy may impair the physical development and functioning of the child or teenager, such as their growth, weight, nutrition, sleep, or puberty. Epilepsy may also influence the physical activity and engagement of the kid or teenager, such as their exercise, sports, or amusement. However, with adequate care, monitoring, and adaptation, children and adolescents living with epilepsy may have a good and active physical existence. They may also benefit from the physical, mental, and social benefits of physical exercise, such as enhanced fitness, mood, cognition, and self-esteem. Some of the strategies to enhance physical health and exercise for children and adolescents living with epilepsy are:

1- Following the medical advice and treatment plan for epilepsy and its management, including monitoring the seizure frequency, severity, and response to medicines.

2- Having a regular and balanced diet, and avoiding any foods or beverages that may cause or aggravate seizures, such as coffee, alcohol, or artificial sweeteners.

3- Having a regular and enough sleep, and avoiding any circumstances that may disturb or impair sleep, such as stress, noise, or light.

4- Having regular and appropriate physical exercise, and picking activities that complement the kid or adolescent's interests, talents, and aspirations.

5- Having a preparticipation assessment and a personalized epilepsy management plan for physical activity, and discussing it with the physical education instructors, coaches, and other personnel.

6- Having a safe and supportive environment for physical exercise, and utilizing any appropriate equipment, adjustments, or measures to avoid or limit the risk of injury or damage.

CHAPTER 6

Epilepsy is a disorder that affects the brain and produces recurring seizures. Seizures are short periods of aberrant electrical activity in the brain that may alter a person's consciousness, movement, feelings, emotions, or behavior. Epilepsy may have different causes, such as hereditary factors, brain damage, infection, or stroke. Epilepsy may also influence a person's learning, memory, temperament, and social skills.

Epilepsy may occur at any age, although it is more frequent in children and older individuals. According to the Centers for Disease Control and Prevention, about 1.2% of people in the United States have active epilepsy, which means they have a history of doctor-diagnosed epilepsy or seizure disorder and are currently taking medication to control it or had one or more seizures in the past year. Epilepsy in older persons is frequently caused by other neurological diseases, such as stroke, brain tumor, infection, or Alzheimer's disease. Epilepsy in older persons brings extra obstacles in treatment and management, such as age-related disorders, usage of other drugs, risk of falls and accidents, and loss of independence.

Epilepsy is diagnosed if a person has experienced at least two unprovoked seizures at least 24 hours apart. Unprovoked seizures do not have an obvious cause, such as fever, low blood sugar, or alcohol withdrawal. Seizures are defined as either focal or generalized, depending on how and where the brain activity triggering the seizure starts. Focal seizures impact just one section of the brain, whereas generalized seizures involve both sides of the brain. Seizures may induce numerous symptoms, such as brief bewilderment, staring spell, rigid muscles, involuntary jerking motions, loss of consciousness, or psychiatric issues.

 The primary therapy for epilepsy is medication, which may diminish or halt seizures in most patients. However, some individuals may not react well to medicine, or may develop negative effects or combinations with other treatments. In certain circumstances, surgery, gadgets, or nutritional treatment may be utilized to treat epilepsy. The choice of therapy relies on various aspects, such as the kind and frequency of seizures, the origin of epilepsy, the age and general health of the individual, and the personal preferences and objectives of the person.

Techniques to manage with epilepsy and enhance the quality of life

Living with epilepsy may be tough, but it is possible to live a pleasant and meaningful life with epilepsy. Some of the techniques to manage with epilepsy and enhance the quality of life are:

1- Seeking and acquiring accurate and up-to-date information regarding epilepsy and its treatment, and sharing it with family, friends, and others who may need to know.

2- Communicating and cooperating with the health care providers and other professionals engaged in the care and support of the person with epilepsy.

3- Seeking and gaining emotional and practical help from many sources, such as counselors, social workers, support groups, or internet forums.

4- Balancing the requirements and obligations of the person with epilepsy with the other parts of life, such as job, education, hobbies, and relationships.

5- Following the medical advice and treatment plan for epilepsy and its management, including monitoring the seizure frequency, severity, and response to therapy.

6- Having a regular and healthy lifestyle, such as eating regularly, sleeping well, exercising moderately, and avoiding stress, alcohol, or other causes of seizures.

7- Having a seizure action plan and a seizure first aid kit, and understanding what to do before, during, and after a seizure.

8- Having a safe and supportive environment, and employing any appropriate equipment, adaptations, or measures to avoid or limit the risk of damage or harm.

Epilepsy is a disorder that affects the brain and produces frequent seizures. Seizures are abrupt bursts of electrical activity in the brain that may alter a person's consciousness, actions, feelings, or emotions. Epilepsy may occur at any age, although it is more frequent in older persons. In fact, epilepsy is the most frequent neurological condition in persons over 65 years old.

There are numerous probable causes of epilepsy in older persons, such as stroke, brain tumor, head injury, Alzheimer's disease, or other brain illnesses. Sometimes, the reason is unknown. Epilepsy in older persons may have distinct symptoms and complications than in younger people. For example, seizures in older persons may be more mild and difficult to notice, such as disorientation, memory lapses, wandering, or dizziness. These symptoms may be misinterpreted for indicators of aging, dementia, or other health conditions

.

Epilepsy may influence the quality of life and independence of older persons. It may raise the risk of falls, fractures, depression, and cognitive deterioration. It may also interfere with driving, social activities, and medication administration. Therefore, it is vital to detect and treat epilepsy in older persons as soon as feasible. The treatment of epilepsy in older persons may entail anti-seizure medicines, surgery, or other therapy. However, the therapy may also bring certain obstacles, such as adverse effects, medication combinations, or compliance concerns. Therefore, it is crucial to work closely with a health care practitioner and an epilepsy expert to determine the appropriate treatment choice for each person .

Epilepsy is a common and curable illness that may afflict older persons. By identifying the indications of seizures, receiving medical assistance, and following the treatment plan, older persons with epilepsy may improve their health and well-being.

CHAPTER 7

Epilepsy and family managing with contraception, pregnancy and menopause in epileptic patients

- Contraception:

Women with epilepsy may use any type of contraception, however certain anti-epileptic medicines (AEDs) may interact with hormonal contraceptives and diminish their efficacy or raise the risk of seizures. The most prevalent AEDs that may disrupt hormonal contraception include carbamazepine, oxcarbazepine, phenytoin, phenobarbital, primidone, and topiramate. Women who use these AEDs should use a greater amount of estrogen in their contraceptive pills, patches, or rings, or consider utilizing non-hormonal options such as condoms, intrauterine devices (IUDs), or sterilization. Valproate is an AED that must not be used in women of reproductive age unless there is a pregnancy prevention program (PPP) in place, since it may cause major birth abnormalities and developmental issues in the unborn infant.

- Pregnancy : Women with epilepsy should also be informed of the potential difficulties during labor and delivery, such as increased risk of seizures, hemorrhage, and fetal distress. They should discuss their birth plan with their physicians and midwives, and have continuous monitoring of the baby's heart rate throughout labor. They should also avoid some pain management measures that might reduce the seizure threshold, such as pethidine and tramadol. After birth, women with epilepsy should continue to take their AEDs as prescribed, and seek advice on nursing, since certain AEDs may transfer into breast milk and damage the infant .

- Menopause:
Women with epilepsy may have changes in their seizure patterns and AED levels throughout menopause, owing to hormonal variations and slower clearance of certain AEDs . They may also experience increased menopausal symptoms, such as hot flashes, mood swings, sleeplessness, and osteoporosis, which may compromise their quality of life and seizure control . Women with epilepsy should visit their physicians about the optimal treatment of their menopause, and examine the advantages and hazards of hormone replacement therapy (HRT), which may assist with menopausal symptoms but may interact with certain AEDs . They should also undergo frequent bone density examinations and take calcium and vitamin D supplements to avoid osteoporosis .

Parenting by persons with epilepsy is an issue that may affect many people who have epilepsy or are hoping to have children. Epilepsy may not preclude individuals from having parents, although it may offer certain obstacles and necessitate some precautions. Here is a note on some of the challenges and recommendations linked to parenting by persons with epilepsy.

- Safety: One of the primary worries for parents with epilepsy is how to keep their children safe during a seizure. Depending on the kind and frequency of seizures, parents may need to take certain additional steps to prevent the risk of damage or harm to themselves or their children. Some of these steps include:
* Dressing, changing, feeding and washing the kid on the floor or in a low position, to prevent falls or drops.
    * Using a cushioned carrycot, sling, pram or stroller to move the kid, rather than carrying them in the arms.
    * Using a wrist strap or a brake on the pram or stroller, to prevent it from rolling away.
    * Keeping the youngster in a safe playpen or childproof room, particularly while alone or experiencing a seizure coming on.
    * Wearing a medical ID bracelet or carrying an ID card, to receive help in case of a seizure in public.

- **Communication:** Another crucial component of parenting by persons with epilepsy is how to speak with their children about their disease. Children may frequently be taught at an early age what to do if their parent has a seizure, such as remaining with them, obtaining aid from someone else, or assisting them themselves. Parents may also explain to their children what epilepsy is, how it affects them, and how they manage it. This may assist the children to comprehend, cope and support their parents better.

- **Lifestyle:** Parenting may be hard and taxing for anybody, but particularly for those with epilepsy, who may have greater trouble obtaining adequate sleep, rest and relaxation. These circumstances may also cause or intensify seizures, thus it is crucial for parents with epilepsy to take care of their health and well-being. Some of the methods to achieve this include:
 * Planning ahead and being prepared for various circumstances and crises.
   * Seeking and accepting support from family, friends, neighbors or professionals, when required.
   * Following the advise of their doctor and taking their prescription consistently and on time.
   * Avoiding or minimizing other possible seizure triggers, such as alcohol, coffee, narcotics, flashing lights or dehydration.
   * Finding time for hobbies, interests, exercise and social activities, to relieve stress and boost mood.

Parenting by persons with epilepsy may be gratifying and enjoyable, as well as stressful and demanding. By taking certain measures, talking freely, and looking after themselves, parents with epilepsy may offer a safe, supportive and caring environment for their children.

CHAPTER 8

Employment and military service for epileptic sufferers.

Epilepsy is a neurological illness where recurring, spontaneous seizures harm you. These seizures are indications of abrupt electrical disruptions in the brain.

To serve in the military, you must fulfill stringent health criteria, which include extensive physical and mental fitness exams meant to ensure service members are able to train, deploy, and confront the difficulties of military tasks.

A number of medical problems, including epilepsy, may disqualify you from serving to guarantee that all military members are capable of withstanding the pressures and demands of service without excessive danger to themselves or others.

According to the U.S. Department of Defense, the military discriminates against persons with epilepsy because it wants military members to be ready for international deployment at any time and with minimal constraints.

- The rules say that an applicant shall be evaluated on an individual basis if there has been no seizure recurrence since age five, or the applicant has been seizure-free without medication for the five years immediately before the application.

- The military may be more flexible regarding pharmaceutical usage if someone is already in the service and has a disease such as epilepsy. Regulations state that an individual will be separated upon developing convulsive disorders, when seizures are not adequately controlled (complete freedom from seizure of any type) by standard drugs which are relatively nontoxic and which do not require frequent clinical and laboratory re-evaluation.

- The UK Armed Forces have similar regulations addressing epilepsy. If you have just experienced a seizure, you are normally degraded for 18 months. You may also be limited in driving and handling firearms. If you have had more than one seizure you are typically regarded unsuited for any trade in the Armed Forces.

- People who have been refused admittance into the military forces based on their history of epilepsy may seek to protest their exclusion by writing to their political representatives since they may be in the greatest position to influence change.

- Employment concerns are responsible for 85% of the expense of epilepsy in society. In the United States, the median income for persons with epilepsy is 93% that of all people.

- People with epilepsy may suffer prejudice, stigma, and difficulties in employment. However, there are several regulations and programs that protect those with disabilities and assist them obtain and retain work.

Epilepsy is a neurological illness that affects the brain and generates seizures, which are abrupt bursts of aberrant electrical activity. Seizures may vary in nature, frequency, and intensity, and can affect various portions of the body and awareness.

People with epilepsy may experience different issues in their everyday life, such as stigma, prejudice, loneliness, anxiety, sadness, memory problems, learning difficulties, and physical injuries . They may also worry about their safety, independence, relationships, education, work, and future .

As a supporter of someone with epilepsy, you may play a significant part in helping them manage with their disease and enhance their quality of life. Here are some ways you may assist them:

1- Understand and sympathize with their situation: Learn as much as you can about epilepsy and how it affects your loved one . Ask them how they feel and what they need from you. Listen to them without criticizing or interfering. Respect their emotions and decisions. Show them that you care and that you are there for them.

2- Provide emotional and practical support: Encourage them to pursue their objectives and interests, and join them in activities they like . Help them identify and access resources and services that may help them, such as medical treatment, counseling, support groups, and legal assistance . Help them with chores that may be difficult or unsafe for them, such as driving, cooking, or handling money . However, do not overprotect them or regard them as helpless or dependent. Allow them to have some control and authority over their life .

3- Help them during and after a seizure: Know the signs and symptoms of their seizures, and how to react to them safely and efficiently . Stay cool and reassure them. Protect children from damage by eliminating any dangerous things or cushioning their head. Loosen any tight garments around their neck. Turn them on their side if they are not breathing properly or have anything in their mouth. Do not restrict them or put anything in their mouth. Time the seizure and call for emergency treatment if it lasts more than five minutes or if they experience repeated seizures . After the seizure, check their respiration and pulse, and treat any injuries. Help them relax and heal in a nice and peaceful area. Stay with them until they are completely aware and oriented .

4 - Handle any obstacles or conflicts: Be patient and flexible with your loved one, since they may experience mood swings, impatience, or violence due to their health or medicine . Communicate with them freely and honestly, and settle any concerns or conflicts gently and politely . Seek professional aid or mediation if required. Do not blame them or yourself for their epilepsy or seizures. Remember that you are both trying your best to manage a complicated and unexpected disease .

5- Take care of yourself and your well-being:
Supporting someone with epilepsy may be gratifying, but sometimes stressful and draining . You may feel many emotions, such as fear, wrath, guilt, grief, or irritation. You may also disregard your own needs and interests, or feel alienated or overwhelmed . Therefore, it is crucial to care for yourself and your health.
Here are some recommendations for self-care:

1- Manage your stress: Find healthy methods to deal with stress, such as exercise, meditation, hobbies, or relaxation techniques . Avoid or restrict alcohol, smoke, caffeine, and drugs . Seek assistance from a therapist or counselor if you feel sad, nervous, or suicidal .

2 - Maintain your physical health: Eat a balanced diet, drink lots of water, get adequate sleep and relax . See your doctor frequently and follow their recommendations. Take any medicine as recommended. Treat any infections or injuries quickly .

3- Nurture your social and emotional health: Spend time with family and friends who support you and make you happy . Join a support group or online community for those who care for someone with epilepsy . Share your thoughts and experiences with those who understand. Seek and accept aid from others when you need it. Do not be scared to ask for favors or help. You do not have to accomplish everything by yourself .

4- Pursue your own goals and passions: Do not lose up on your hopes and aspirations because of your loved one's epilepsy . Continue to work, study, or volunteer, if feasible and desired. Engage in things that provide you pleasure and contentment, such as sports, arts, music, or travel . Set reasonable and achievable objectives for yourself, and celebrate your successes .

CHAPTER 9

Legal and financial issues in epilepsy

People with epilepsy are a vulnerable population who frequently experience prejudice and stigma in different areas of their life, including as health, education, work, housing, and social involvement. However, persons with epilepsy have the same human rights as anybody else, and they are allowed to enjoy them without any restrictions or limits. There are various laws and regulations at the national and international levels that protect and promote the rights of individuals with epilepsy, and that strive to secure their full inclusion and engagement in society.

One of the most significant legal mechanisms that safeguard the rights of individuals with epilepsy is the Convention on the Rights of Persons with Disabilities (CRPD), which was accepted by the United Nations in 2006 and went into effect in 2008. The CRPD is a comprehensive and enforceable convention that includes a broad variety of rights and duties for state parties, such as non-discrimination, accessibility, reasonable accommodation, health, education, job, social protection, and participation in public and political life. The CRPD acknowledges that individuals with disabilities, including those with epilepsy, are subjects of rights and not objects of charity, and that they have the right to make their own judgments and choices about their life. The CRPD also provides a monitoring system, formed of a Committee of experts and a Conference of States Parties, to supervise the implementation of the Convention and to hear complaints from individuals or groups of persons who claim to be victims of a breach of the Convention.

Another major legal document that protects the rights of individuals with epilepsy is the International Covenant on Economic, Social and Cultural Rights (ICESCR), which was ratified by the United Nations in 1966 and went into effect in 1976. The ICESCR is a binding treaty that affirms the right of everyone to enjoy the highest the right to freedom of speech, the right to freedom of assembly and association, and the right to non-discrimination, among others. The ECHR also established a monitoring body, constituted of a Court of Human Rights, to accept and resolve complaints from people or groups of persons who claim to be victims of a breach of the Convention.

In Africa, the African Charter on Human and Peoples' Rights (ACHPR), which was adopted by the Organization of African Unity in 1981 and entered into force in 1986, affirms the right to dignity, the right to equality, the right to health, the right to education, the right to work, the right to social and economic development, and the right to participate in the cultural life of the community, among others. The ACHPR also establishes a monitoring mechanism, composed of a Commission and a Court of Human and Peoples' Rights, to examine the reports submitted by states parties on the measures they have taken to implement the Charter and to receive and decide on complaints from individuals or groups of individuals who claim to be victims of a violation of the Charter.

At the national level, there are numerous laws and policies that protect and promote the rights of persons with epilepsy, depending on the country and the situation. Some examples are:

- In the United States, the Americans with Disabilities Act (ADA), which was enacted in 1990 and amended in 2008, prohibits discrimination against individuals with disabilities in all areas of public life, such as employment, education, transportation, and access to public and private places and services. The ADA also compels employers, governmental bodies, and private enterprises to make reasonable accommodations to those with disabilities, unless it would create undue hardship. The ADA includes persons with epilepsy, as long as their illness severely impairs one or more key living activities.

- In India, the Rights of Persons with Disabilities Act, 2016, which supersedes the old Persons with Disabilities (Equal Opportunities, Protection of Rights and Full Participation) Act, 1995, and tries to harmonize with the requirements of the CRPD. The Act recognizes

21 types of disabilities, including epilepsy, and grants them various rights and entitlements, such as reservation in education, employment, and political representation, accessibility to public buildings and transport, social security and health care, and legal capacity and guardianship.

- In Ghana, the Individuals with Disability Act, 2006 (Act 715), which intends to provide for the rights, protection and management of individuals with disability, and to create a National Council on Persons with Disability. The Act outlaws discrimination against individuals with disabilities in numerous spheres, including education, work, health, transportation, and access to public places and services. The Act also allows for the creation of a Disability Fund to assist the welfare and rehabilitation of individuals with disability.

These are some of the legal rights of persons with epilepsy in various regions of the globe. However, it is crucial to highlight that possessing legal rights does not always guarantee that they are recognized and enforced in reality. There are still numerous problems and hurdles that persons with epilepsy experience in their everyday lives, such as lack of knowledge, stigma, discrimination, misinformation, and lack of resources. Therefore, there is a need for more advocacy, education, and empowerment of people with epilepsy and their families, as well as more collaboration and coordination among different stakeholders, such as governments, civil society, health professionals, and international organizations, to ensure that the rights of people with epilepsy are realized and protected.

Insurance and government aid

Epilepsy is a neurological condition that causes recurring seizures. People with epilepsy may have difficulty in acquiring inexpensive and adequate health coverage and treatment. Depending on their position, people may have various alternatives for insurance and government help.

One alternative is the Affordable Care Act (ACA), which established the Marketplaces where customers may purchase individual or family insurance plans with subsidies to help cut the cost. The ACA also includes various insurance changes, such as barring insurers from rejecting coverage or charging extra to those with pre-existing diseases like epilepsy, and abolishing lifetime and yearly restrictions on coverage. The ACA also provided states the choice to expand their Medicaid programs, which provide healthcare for low-income Americans, including one third of those with epilepsy. Medicaid covers a variety of services, including doctor visits, hospital stays, prescription medicines, and long-term care.

Another alternative is Medicare, which offers health insurance for Americans age 65 and older, and to younger persons with disabilities[2]. Medicare covers hospital care, medical services, and prescription medicines, but it may not pay all the expenses of epilepsy treatment. People with Medicare may also participate in Medicare Advantage plans, which are provided by private organizations and may offer extra benefits, such as vision, dental, and hearing care[2].

People with epilepsy may potentially qualify for Social Security Disability Insurance (SSDI) or Supplemental Security Income (SSI), or both, provided they fulfill specific standards. SSDI is a program that gives benefits to persons who have worked and paid Social Security taxes, but are unable to work due to a disability. SSI is a program that distributes benefits to persons who have minimal income and resources, and are handicapped, blind, or old. Both programs contain medical standards that evaluate whether a person's epilepsy is severe enough to qualify as a disability. People who receive SSDI or SSI may also be eligible for Medicaid or Medicare.

There are also various nonprofit organizations that may help persons with epilepsy identify and apply for patient assistance programs, which are sponsored by medication makers to provide free or low-cost medicines to those who cannot afford them. Some of these organizations include NeedyMeds.Org, Medicine Assistance Tool, PatientAsisstance.com, RxAsslst,

Veteran's Affairs, Rx Outreach, and FamilyWize
Community Service Partnership.

People with epilepsy may also contact their local
Epilepsy Foundation to acquire additional information
and help on health coverage and care. The Epilepsy
Foundation also campaigns for legislation that increases
access and cost of epilepsy treatment and services.

CHAPTER 10

Antiepileptic drugs and their effects

Antiepileptic medicines are pharmaceuticals that are used to treat epileptic seizures, which are abnormal electrical activity in the brain that may induce convulsions, loss of consciousness, or other symptoms. Antiepileptic medications act by lowering the excitability of the neurons, stopping them from firing excessively or spreading the seizure to other areas of the brain.

There are many distinct kinds of antiepileptic medications, and they have varied modes of action, adverse effects, and interactions. Some of the most prevalent antiepileptic medications are:

- **Carbamazepine (Tegretol):** This medicine inhibits sodium channels, which are important in the transmission of nerve impulses. It is useful for partial and generalized seizures, although it might aggravate certain kinds of epilepsy, particularly in youngsters. It may also interact with many other medicines, such as antibiotics, antifungals, antidepressants, and oral contraceptives.

- **Valproate (Depakote):** This medicine boosts the levels of a neurotransmitter called gamma-aminobutyric acid (GABA), which suppresses the activity of neurons. It is used for several forms of seizures, including absence seizures, which cause momentary gaps of consciousness. It may also be used to treat bipolar disorder and migraine headaches. However, it may cause major adverse effects, including liver damage, pancreatitis, weight gain, and birth abnormalities.

- **Lamotrigine (Lamictal):** This medicine similarly inhibits sodium channels, although in a different manner than carbamazepine. It is used for partial and generalized seizures, as well as Lennox-Gastaut syndrome, which is a severe type of epilepsy that originates in infancy. It may also be used to treat bipolar disorder. It has a lesser risk of interactions than carbamazepine, but it may induce a rare but possibly deadly skin response called Stevens-Johnson syndrome.

- **Levetiracetam (Keppra):** This medicine has a unique mode of action that is not entirely known, although it may include binding to a protein called synaptic vesicle protein 2A (SV2A), which is involved in the release of neurotransmitters. It is utilized for partial and generalized seizures, as well as myoclonic seizures, which involve abrupt jerks of the muscles. It has a minimal risk of interactions and adverse effects, although it might induce mood changes, irritation, and sadness.

These are only a few examples of antiepileptic medicines, and there are many more that have various advantages and cons. The choice of antiepileptic treatment relies on several aspects, such as the kind and frequency of seizures, the age and medical history of the patient, the possible adverse effects and interactions, and the cost and availability of the drug. Antiepileptic medicines should be given by a doctor who specializes in epilepsy, and the dose and frequency should be changed according to the patient's reaction and blood levels. Antiepileptic medicines may help control seizures, but they do not cure epilepsy, and they may have to be used for life.

Ketogenic diet for epilepsy and how to prepare it

The ketogenic diet is a particular high-fat, low-carbohydrate diet that helps to manage seizures in certain persons with epilepsy. It is generally used in children with seizures that do not respond to drugs, but it may also aid some adults with epilepsy. The diet works by altering the way the brain absorbs energy from the food we consume. Normally, the brain utilizes glucose (a form of sugar) as its major fuel source, but when carbs are limited, the body breaks down fat into ketone bodies, which may substitute glucose as the brain's fuel. This condition of ketosis may lessen the frequency and severity of seizures by changing the amounts of specific neurotransmitters in the brain, such as glutamate and GABA, which are implicated in seizure activity. The diet may help lower inflammation in the brain, which may provoke seizures in certain situations.

The ketogenic diet is not a standard diet that can be followed by everybody. It involves careful planning and supervision by a team of medical specialists, including a neurologist and a dietician. The diet is quite stringent and accurate, and it requires measuring and weighing the meal amounts and tracking the calories, fluids, and ratios of fat, protein, and carbohydrate. The diet may also involve taking vitamin and mineral supplements to avoid deficits. The diet may have various negative effects, such as constipation, dehydration, kidney stones, high cholesterol, and weight loss or increase. Therefore, it is necessary to follow the diet as suggested and to have frequent blood tests and check-ups to evaluate the health and seizure control of the individual on the diet.

To start the ketogenic diet, the individual may need to fast for a brief amount of time (typically 18 to 24 hours) to induce ketosis quicker. This may be done in the hospital or at home under medical supervision. Then, the diet is progressively introduced by increasing the calories and the fat to carbohydrate and protein ratio over a few days. The average ratio for the basic ketogenic diet is 4:1, which implies 4 grams of fat for every 1 gram of protein and carbohydrate combined. This indicates that around 90% of the calories come from fat, 6% from protein, and 4% from carbohydrates. However, there are many varieties of the ketogenic diet, such as the modified Atkins diet, the medium-chain triglyceride (MCT) diet, and the low glycemic index treatment (LGIT), which may have differing ratios and greater freedom in food choices. The optimal sort of ketogenic diet for each person depends on their specific requirements, tastes, and tolerance.

To prepare the ketogenic diet, the individual will need to use a food scale and measuring cups and spoons to weigh and measure the meal quantities precisely. The dish should be made using high-fat foods, such as butter, cream, oil, mayonnaise, cheese, and nuts. The meal should also be low in carbohydrate, which includes avoiding or restricting items such as bread, pasta, rice, cereal, fruits, vegetables, milk, yogurt, and sweets. The meal should give enough protein for optimal growth and development, but not too much, since excess protein might interfere with ketosis. The diet should also offer enough fluids to avoid dehydration, but not too much, since additional fluids might dilute the ketones in the blood. The diet should be split into three or four meals each day, and snacking should be avoided or reduced. The meal should be consumed slowly and fully, and any leftovers should be discarded.

Here is an example meal for one day on the traditional ketogenic diet with a 4:1 ratio:

Breakfast:
- Scrambled eggs (prepared with 2 eggs, 36 g of butter, and 9 g of cream)
- Bacon (14 g)
- Water or unsweetened tea or coffee

Lunch:
- Tuna salad (prepared with 28 g of tuna, 14 g of mayonnaise, and 3 g of celery)
- Lettuce (7 g) with ranch dressing (14 g)
- Water or unsweetened tea or coffee

Dinner:
- Chicken (28 g) with Alfredo sauce (28 g)
- Broccoli (14 g) with butter (14 g)
- Water or unsweetened tea or coffee

Dessert:
- Whipped cream (28 g) with strawberries (7 g)

The ketogenic diet for epilepsy is a sophisticated and hard diet that needs medical advice and assistance. It is not a cure for epilepsy, but it may help some patients achieve improved seizure control and quality of life. Whether you are interested in attempting the ketogenic diet for epilepsy, you should consult your doctor and dietitian first to establish whether it is acceptable and safe for you.

CONCLUSION

Epilepsy is a complex and challenging condition that affects millions of people worldwide. It can cause various types of seizures, which can have a significant impact on the quality of life of the patients and their families. However, with proper diagnosis, treatment and support, many people with epilepsy can lead fulfilling and productive lives. In this book, Dr Jacob Jabin, a renowned neurologist and epilepsy expert, provides a comprehensive and practical guide on epilepsy for patients, families and caregivers. He covers topics such as the causes, types, symptoms, diagnosis, treatment and management of epilepsy, as well as the psychosocial, legal and ethical aspects of living with epilepsy. He also offers tips and advice on how to cope with common challenges, such as stigma, discrimination, education, employment, driving, pregnancy and parenting. He also shares inspiring stories of people who have overcome epilepsy and achieved their goals and dreams. This book is a valuable resource for anyone who wants to learn more about epilepsy and how to live well with it. It is written in a clear and accessible language, with illustrations to enhance understanding. It also includes a glossary of terms, a list of resources and a bibliography for further reading. Epilepsy Guide by Dr Jacob Jabin is a must-read for anyone who wants to gain a better understanding of epilepsy and its implications. It is a book that empowers, educates and encourages people with epilepsy and their loved ones to face epilepsy with confidence and optimism.

www.ingramcontent.com/pod-product-compliance
Lightning Source LLC
Chambersburg PA
CBHW060951260726
48661CB00005B/1833